Thank you for purchasing my book! I truly hope it is a blessing to you!
-Moxie Rae

IF YOU FOUND THIS BOOK HELPFUL FOR YOUR PUMPING JOURNEY, PLEASE LEAVE A REVIEW AND HELP OTHER MAMAS FIND IT TOO! THANK YOU!

Copyright © 2021 Moxie Rae
All Rights Reserved

Dedication

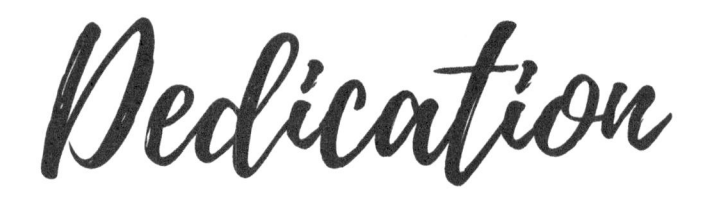

This book is dedicated to my babies. Without them, this book quite literally wouldn't exist. I am so proud to be your Mama! I love you!

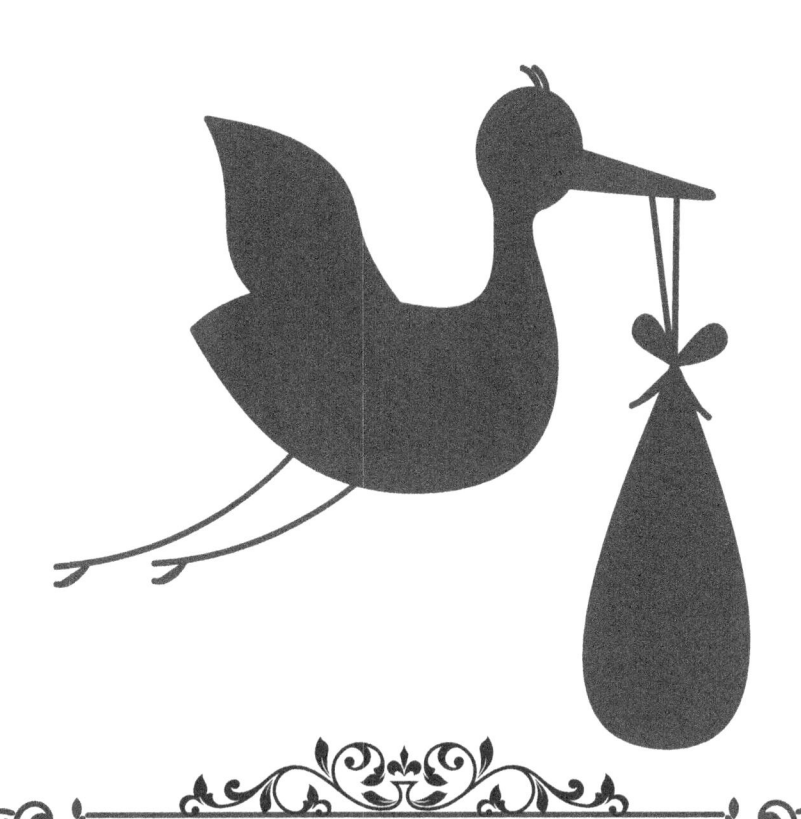

Please note: I created this book out of my own limited knowledge from my experience feeding my two children. I exclusively nursed my first daughter until she was two and a half, and I exclusively pumped for my second daughter until she was a year old. However, please hear me that I am not a lactation consultant and this book is not meant to give health advice or to be taken as such.

Helpful Hints

1. Exclusively pumping is not easy! Make it a little less stressful by having enough sets of pump parts and bottles to only need to wash them once a day.
2. Lay milk bags flat to freeze and then store them in gallon size freezer bags to make milk bricks. Even better if each small bag has the same amount of oz and each brick has the same number of bags. This makes it easy to calculate how much milk is in your stash.
3. Speaking of the freezer, get an alarm to alert you if your deep freezer is too warm.
4. I highly recommend joining Josi Wolfenbarger's group Breast Bottle and Beyond for support. You can find information at www.breastbottleandbeyond.com.
5. Do breast compressions and massage your breasts towards your nipple while pumping to increase your output!

6. The flange from your pump makes a great funnel for filling baby bottles!

7. A pump with a rechargeable battery is worth its weight in gold! If you need to move to get a glass of water or answer the phone, it's great to be able to move more than three feet from the wall outlet! The battery-powered pump also makes pumping in the car or anywhere out of the house much easier.

8. If you feel like you are not getting as much milk at each pump session, check if you need to replace your valves and membranes. Also, make sure you stay hydrated!

9. Pump every 2 hours around the clock for as long as you can to establish a great milk supply. Keep track of your daily total ounces pumped so you know if something you are doing or eating is decreasing your milk supply. Make any changes to your pumping schedule slowly to protect your supply from dropping.

10. Ask for help when you need it! Being able to pump because you choose to, or because your baby cannot nurse for whatever reason, is a huge blessing but it creates a ton of work! I have done both nursing and pumping. In my opinion, pumping creates so much more work! So don't be afraid to ask for help!

Exclusively Pumping Log

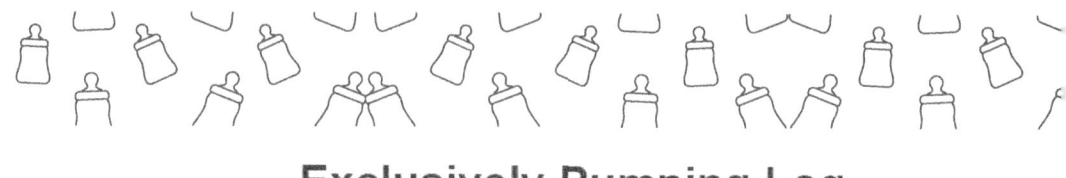

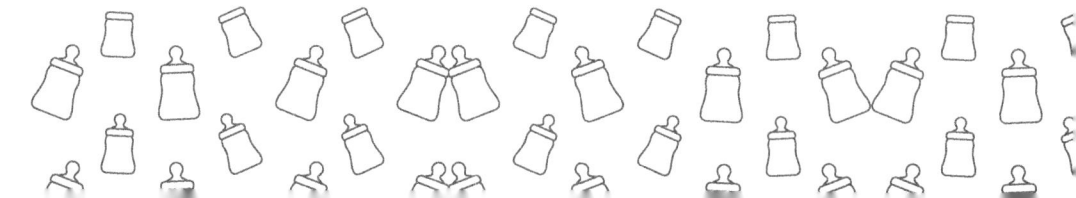

Date: 10/07/2020

Pumping Log

Time of Pump	Amount Pumped
6:00 AM	3 oz
8:00 AM	3 oz
10:10 AM	5.5 oz
12:00 AM	4.25 oz
2:00 PM	3 oz
4:00 PM	2 oz
6:00 PM	2 oz
8:00 PM	3 oz
10:00 PM	2 oz
12:00 AM	3
2:00 AM	8 oz
4:00 AM	3 oz

Total Ounces Pumped: _____ oz

Feeding Log

Time of Feed	Amount Fed
6:30 AM	4 oz
9:00 AM	4 oz
12:00 PM	4 oz
3:00 PM	4 oz
6:00 PM	4 oz
9:00 PM	4 oz
12:00 AM	4 oz
3:00 AM	4 oz

Total Ounces Fed: __32__ oz

Amount in the freezer at the start of the day: ___208___ oz
Amount thawed to feed the baby today: -- ___32___ oz
Amount added to the freezer today: + ___40___ oz
Amount in freezer stash at the end of the day: = ___216___ oz

Notes: _Baby was pretty gassy today. I had extra dairy the day I pumped the milk she drank so she may be having a hard time digesting lactose._

Today I had eggs at breakfast.

Exclusively Pumping Log

Date: ___/___/___

Pumping Log		Feeding Log	
Time of Pump	Amount Pumped	Time of Feed	Amount Fed
Total Ounces Pumped: _____ oz		Total Ounces Fed: _____ oz	

Amount in the freezer at the start of the day: _____ oz
Amount thawed to feed the baby today: -- _____ oz
Amount added to the freezer today: + _____ oz
Amount in freezer stash at the end of the day: = _____ oz

Notes: _____
_____
_____
_____
_____
_____

Exclusively Pumping Log

Date: ___/___/___

Pumping Log			Feeding Log	
Time of Pump	Amount Pumped		Time of Feed	Amount Fed
Total Ounces Pumped: _____ oz			Total Ounces Fed: _____ oz	

Amount in the freezer at the start of the day: _____ oz
Amount thawed to feed the baby today: − _____ oz
Amount added to the freezer today: + _____ oz
Amount in freezer stash at the end of the day: = _____ oz

Notes: _____
_____
_____
_____
_____
_____
_____
_____

Exclusively Pumping Log

Date: ___/___/___

Pumping Log	
Time of Pump	Amount Pumped
Total Ounces Pumped: _____ oz	

Feeding Log	
Time of Feed	Amount Fed
Total Ounces Fed: _____ oz	

Amount in the freezer at the start of the day: _____ oz
Amount thawed to feed the baby today: -_____ oz
Amount added to the freezer today: +_____ oz
Amount in freezer stash at the end of the day: =_____ oz

Notes: _____
_____
_____
_____
_____
_____
_____

Exclusively Pumping Log

Date: ___/___/___

Pumping Log ||	Feeding Log	
Time of Pump	Amount Pumped	Time of Feed	Amount Fed
Total Ounces Pumped: _____ oz		Total Ounces Fed: _____ oz	

Amount in the freezer at the start of the day: _____ oz
Amount thawed to feed the baby today: -- _____ oz
Amount added to the freezer today: + _____ oz
Amount in freezer stash at the end of the day: = _____ oz

Notes: _____
_____
_____
_____
_____
_____
_____

Exclusively Pumping Log

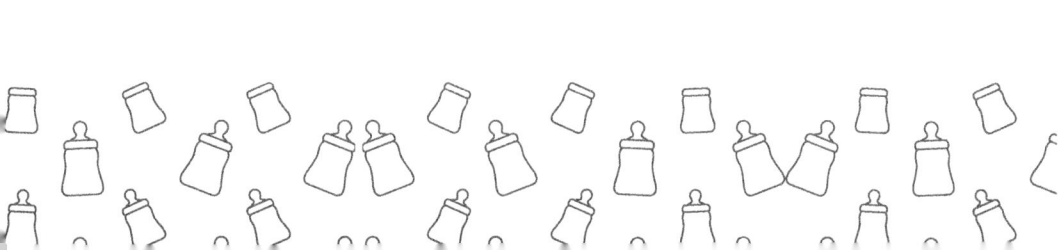

Date: ___/___/___

Pumping Log		Feeding Log	
Time of Pump	Amount Pumped	Time of Feed	Amount Fed
Total Ounces Pumped: _____ oz		Total Ounces Fed: _____ oz	

Amount in the freezer at the start of the day: _____ oz
Amount thawed to feed the baby today: -- _____ oz
Amount added to the freezer today: + _____ oz
Amount in freezer stash at the end of the day: = _____ oz

Notes: _____
_____
_____
_____
_____
_____
_____
_____

Exclusively Pumping Log

Date: __/__/__

Pumping Log	
Time of Pump	Amount Pumped
Total Ounces Pumped: _____ oz	

Feeding Log	
Time of Feed	Amount Fed
Total Ounces Fed: _____ oz	

Amount in the freezer at the start of the day: _____ oz
Amount thawed to feed the baby today: -- _____ oz
Amount added to the freezer today: + _____ oz
Amount in freezer stash at the end of the day: = _____ oz

Notes: _____
_____
_____
_____
_____
_____
_____
_____

Exclusively Pumping Log

Date: ___/___/___

Pumping Log	
Time of Pump	Amount Pumped
Total Ounces Pumped: _____ oz	

Feeding Log	
Time of Feed	Amount Fed
Total Ounces Fed: _____ oz	

Amount in the freezer at the start of the day: _____ oz
Amount thawed to feed the baby today: -- _____ oz
Amount added to the freezer today: + _____ oz
Amount in freezer stash at the end of the day: = _____ oz

Notes: _____
_____
_____
_____
_____
_____
_____

Exclusively Pumping Log

Date:___/___/___

Pumping Log		Feeding Log	
Time of Pump	Amount Pumped	Time of Feed	Amount Fed
Total Ounces Pumped: _____ oz		Total Ounces Fed: _____ oz	

Amount in the freezer at the start of the day: _____ oz
Amount thawed to feed the baby today: − _____ oz
Amount added to the freezer today: + _____ oz
Amount in freezer stash at the end of the day: = _____ oz

Notes: _____
_____
_____
_____
_____
_____
_____

Exclusively Pumping Log

Date: ___/___/___

Pumping Log		Feeding Log	
Time of Pump	Amount Pumped	Time of Feed	Amount Fed
Total Ounces Pumped: _____ oz		Total Ounces Fed: _____ oz	

Amount in the freezer at the start of the day: _____ oz
Amount thawed to feed the baby today: -- _____ oz
Amount added to the freezer today: + _____ oz
Amount in freezer stash at the end of the day: = _____ oz

Notes: _____
_____
_____
_____
_____
_____
_____

Exclusively Pumping Log

Date: ___/___/___

Pumping Log		Feeding Log	
Time of Pump	Amount Pumped	Time of Feed	Amount Fed
Total Ounces Pumped: _____ oz		Total Ounces Fed: _____ oz	

Amount in the freezer at the start of the day: _____ oz
Amount thawed to feed the baby today: -- _____ oz
Amount added to the freezer today: + _____ oz
Amount in freezer stash at the end of the day: = _____ oz

Notes: _____
_____
_____
_____
_____
_____
_____

Exclusively Pumping Log

Date: ___/___/___

Pumping Log			Feeding Log	
Time of Pump	Amount Pumped		Time of Feed	Amount Fed
Total Ounces Pumped: _____ oz.			Total Ounces Fed: _____ oz	

Amount in the freezer at the start of the day: _____ oz
Amount thawed to feed the baby today: − _____ oz
Amount added to the freezer today: + _____ oz
Amount in freezer stash at the end of the day: = _____ oz

Notes: _____
_____
_____
_____
_____
_____

Exclusively Pumping Log

Date: ___/___/___

Pumping Log			Feeding Log	
Time of Pump	Amount Pumped		Time of Feed	Amount Fed
Total Ounces Pumped: _____ oz			Total Ounces Fed: _____ oz	

Amount in the freezer at the start of the day: _____ oz
Amount thawed to feed the baby today: −_____ oz
Amount added to the freezer today: +_____ oz
Amount in freezer stash at the end of the day: =_____ oz

Notes: _____
_____
_____
_____
_____
_____
_____

Exclusively Pumping Log

Date: ___/___/___

Pumping Log			Feeding Log	
Time of Pump	Amount Pumped		Time of Feed	Amount Fed
Total Ounces Pumped: _____ oz			Total Ounces Fed: _____ oz	

Amount in the freezer at the start of the day:　　_____ oz
Amount thawed to feed the baby today:　　-- _____ oz
Amount added to the freezer today:　　+ _____ oz
Amount in freezer stash at the end of the day:　　= _____ oz

Notes: _____
_____
_____
_____
_____
_____
_____

Exclusively Pumping Log

Date: ___/___/___

Pumping Log			Feeding Log	
Time of Pump	Amount Pumped		Time of Feed	Amount Fed
Total Ounces Pumped: _____ oz			Total Ounces Fed: _____ oz	

Amount in the freezer at the start of the day: _____ oz
Amount thawed to feed the baby today: − _____ oz
Amount added to the freezer today: + _____ oz
Amount in freezer stash at the end of the day: = _____ oz

Notes: _____
_____
_____
_____
_____
_____
_____
_____

Exclusively Pumping Log

Date: ___/___/___

Pumping Log		Feeding Log	
Time of Pump	Amount Pumped	Time of Feed	Amount Fed
Total Ounces Pumped: _____ oz		Total Ounces Fed: _____ oz	

Amount in the freezer at the start of the day: _____ oz
Amount thawed to feed the baby today: -- _____ oz
Amount added to the freezer today: + _____ oz
Amount in freezer stash at the end of the day: = _____ oz

Notes: _____
_____
_____
_____
_____
_____
_____

Exclusively Pumping Log

Date: ___/___/___

Pumping Log			Feeding Log	
Time of Pump	Amount Pumped	Time of Feed	Amount Fed
Total Ounces Pumped: _____ oz		Total Ounces Fed: _____ oz	

Amount in the freezer at the start of the day: _____ oz
Amount thawed to feed the baby today: -- _____ oz
Amount added to the freezer today: + _____ oz
Amount in freezer stash at the end of the day: = _____ oz

Notes: _____
_____
_____
_____
_____
_____
_____
_____

Exclusively Pumping Log

Date: ___/___/___

Pumping Log			Feeding Log	
Time of Pump	Amount Pumped		Time of Feed	Amount Fed
Total Ounces Pumped: _____ oz			Total Ounces Fed: _____ oz	

Amount in the freezer at the start of the day: _____ oz
Amount thawed to feed the baby today: -- _____ oz
Amount added to the freezer today: + _____ oz
Amount in freezer stash at the end of the day: = _____ oz

Notes: _____
_____
_____
_____
_____
_____
_____
_____

Exclusively Pumping Log

Date: ___/___/___

Pumping Log	
Time of Pump	Amount Pumped

Total Ounces Pumped: _____ oz

Feeding Log	
Time of Feed	Amount Fed

Total Ounces Fed: _____ oz

Amount in the freezer at the start of the day: _____ oz
Amount thawed to feed the baby today: -- _____ oz
Amount added to the freezer today: + _____ oz
Amount in freezer stash at the end of the day: = _____ oz

Notes: _____
_____
_____
_____
_____
_____
_____

Exclusively Pumping Log

Date: ___/___/___

Pumping Log		Feeding Log	
Time of Pump	Amount Pumped	Time of Feed	Amount Fed
Total Ounces Pumped: _____ oz		Total Ounces Fed: _____ oz	

Amount in the freezer at the start of the day: _____ oz
Amount thawed to feed the baby today: -- _____ oz
Amount added to the freezer today: + _____ oz
Amount in freezer stash at the end of the day: = _____ oz

Notes: _____
_____
_____
_____
_____

Exclusively Pumping Log

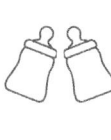

Date: ___/___/___

Pumping Log			Feeding Log	
Time of Pump	Amount Pumped	Time of Feed	Amount Fed
Total Ounces Pumped: _____ oz		Total Ounces Fed: _____ oz	

Amount in the freezer at the start of the day: _____ oz
Amount thawed to feed the baby today: − _____ oz
Amount added to the freezer today: + _____ oz
Amount in freezer stash at the end of the day: = _____ oz

Notes: _____
_____
_____
_____
_____
_____
_____

Exclusively Pumping Log

Date: ___/___/___

Pumping Log			Feeding Log	
Time of Pump	Amount Pumped		Time of Feed	Amount Fed
Total Ounces Pumped: _____ oz			Total Ounces Fed: _____ oz	

Amount in the freezer at the start of the day: _____ oz
Amount thawed to feed the baby today: -- _____ oz
Amount added to the freezer today: + _____ oz
Amount in freezer stash at the end of the day: = _____ oz

Notes: _____
_____
_____
_____
_____
_____
_____
_____

Exclusively Pumping Log

Date: ___/___/___

Pumping Log			Feeding Log	
Time of Pump	Amount Pumped		Time of Feed	Amount Fed

Total Ounces Pumped: _____ oz   Total Ounces Fed: _____ oz

Amount in the freezer at the start of the day: _____ oz
Amount thawed to feed the baby today: -- _____ oz
Amount added to the freezer today: + _____ oz
Amount in freezer stash at the end of the day: = _____ oz

Notes: _____
_____
_____
_____
_____
_____
_____

Exclusively Pumping Log

Date: ___/___/___

Pumping Log		Feeding Log	
Time of Pump	Amount Pumped	Time of Feed	Amount Fed
Total Ounces Pumped: _____ oz		Total Ounces Fed: _____ oz	

Amount in the freezer at the start of the day: _____ oz
Amount thawed to feed the baby today: -- _____ oz
Amount added to the freezer today: + _____ oz
Amount in freezer stash at the end of the day: = _____ oz

Notes: _____
_____
_____
_____
_____
_____

Exclusively Pumping Log

Date: ___/___/___

Pumping Log ||| Feeding Log		
Time of Pump	Amount Pumped	Time of Feed	Amount Fed
Total Ounces Pumped: _____ oz		Total Ounces Fed: _____ oz	

Amount in the freezer at the start of the day: _____ oz
Amount thawed to feed the baby today: − _____ oz
Amount added to the freezer today: + _____ oz
Amount in freezer stash at the end of the day: = _____ oz

Notes: _____
_____
_____
_____
_____
_____
_____

Exclusively Pumping Log

Date: ___/___/___

Pumping Log		Feeding Log	
Time of Pump	Amount Pumped	Time of Feed	Amount Fed
Total Ounces Pumped: _____ oz		Total Ounces Fed: _____ oz	

Amount in the freezer at the start of the day: _____ oz
Amount thawed to feed the baby today: -- _____ oz
Amount added to the freezer today: + _____ oz
Amount in freezer stash at the end of the day: = _____ oz

Notes: _____
_____
_____
_____
_____
_____
_____

Exclusively Pumping Log

Date: __/__/__

Pumping Log		Feeding Log	
Time of Pump	Amount Pumped	Time of Feed	Amount Fed
Total Ounces Pumped: _____ oz		Total Ounces Fed: _____ oz	

Amount in the freezer at the start of the day: _____ oz
Amount thawed to feed the baby today: -- _____ oz
Amount added to the freezer today: + _____ oz
Amount in freezer stash at the end of the day: = _____ oz

Notes: _____
_____
_____
_____
_____
_____
_____

Exclusively Pumping Log

Date: ___/___/___

Pumping Log		Feeding Log	
Time of Pump	Amount Pumped	Time of Feed	Amount Fed
Total Ounces Pumped: _____ oz		Total Ounces Fed: _____ oz	

Amount in the freezer at the start of the day: _____ oz
Amount thawed to feed the baby today: -- _____ oz
Amount added to the freezer today: + _____ oz
Amount in freezer stash at the end of the day: = _____ oz

Notes: _____
_____
_____
_____
_____
_____
_____

Exclusively Pumping Log

Date: __/__/__

Pumping Log		Feeding Log	
Time of Pump	Amount Pumped	Time of Feed	Amount Fed
Total Ounces Pumped: _____ oz		Total Ounces Fed: _____ oz	

Amount in the freezer at the start of the day: _____ oz
Amount thawed to feed the baby today: − _____ oz
Amount added to the freezer today: + _____ oz
Amount in freezer stash at the end of the day: = _____ oz

Notes: _____
_____
_____
_____
_____
_____
_____

Exclusively Pumping Log

Date: __/__/__

Pumping Log		Feeding Log	
Time of Pump	Amount Pumped	Time of Feed	Amount Fed

Total Ounces Pumped: _____ oz   Total Ounces Fed: _____ oz

Amount in the freezer at the start of the day: _____ oz
Amount thawed to feed the baby today: -- _____ oz
Amount added to the freezer today: + _____ oz
Amount in freezer stash at the end of the day: = _____ oz

Notes: _____
_____
_____
_____
_____
_____
_____

Exclusively Pumping Log

Date: ___/___/___

Pumping Log

Time of Pump	Amount Pumped

Total Ounces Pumped: _____ oz

Feeding Log

Time of Feed	Amount Fed

Total Ounces Fed: _____ oz

Amount in the freezer at the start of the day: _____ oz
Amount thawed to feed the baby today: -- _____ oz
Amount added to the freezer today: + _____ oz
Amount in freezer stash at the end of the day: = _____ oz

Notes: _____
_____
_____
_____
_____
_____
_____
_____

Exclusively Pumping Log

Date: ___/___/___

Pumping Log		Feeding Log	
Time of Pump	Amount Pumped	Time of Feed	Amount Fed
Total Ounces Pumped: _____ oz		Total Ounces Fed: _____ oz	

Amount in the freezer at the start of the day: _____ oz
Amount thawed to feed the baby today: -- _____ oz
Amount added to the freezer today: + _____ oz
Amount in freezer stash at the end of the day: = _____ oz

Notes: _____
_____
_____
_____
_____
_____

Exclusively Pumping Log

Date: ___/___/___

Pumping Log			Feeding Log	
Time of Pump	Amount Pumped		Time of Feed	Amount Fed
Total Ounces Pumped: _____ oz			Total Ounces Fed: _____ oz	

Amount in the freezer at the start of the day: _____ oz
Amount thawed to feed the baby today: −_____ oz
Amount added to the freezer today: +_____ oz
Amount in freezer stash at the end of the day: =_____ oz

Notes: _____
_____
_____
_____
_____
_____
_____

Exclusively Pumping Log

Date: ___/___/___

Pumping Log			Feeding Log	
Time of Pump	Amount Pumped		Time of Feed	Amount Fed
Total Ounces Pumped: _____ oz			Total Ounces Fed: _____ oz	

Amount in the freezer at the start of the day: _____ oz
Amount thawed to feed the baby today: -- _____ oz
Amount added to the freezer today: + _____ oz
Amount in freezer stash at the end of the day: = _____ oz

Notes: _____
_____
_____
_____
_____
_____
_____

Exclusively Pumping Log

Date: ___/___/___

Pumping Log

Time of Pump	Amount Pumped
Total Ounces Pumped: _____ oz	

Feeding Log

Time of Feed	Amount Fed
Total Ounces Fed: _____ oz	

Amount in the freezer at the start of the day: _____ oz
Amount thawed to feed the baby today: −_____ oz
Amount added to the freezer today: +_____ oz
Amount in freezer stash at the end of the day: =_____ oz

Notes: _____
_____
_____
_____
_____
_____
_____

Exclusively Pumping Log

Date: ___/___/___

Pumping Log			Feeding Log	
Time of Pump	Amount Pumped		Time of Feed	Amount Fed
Total Ounces Pumped: _____ oz			Total Ounces Fed: _____ oz	

Amount in the freezer at the start of the day: _____ oz
Amount thawed to feed the baby today: −_____ oz
Amount added to the freezer today: +_____ oz
Amount in freezer stash at the end of the day: =_____ oz

Notes: _____
_____
_____
_____
_____
_____

Exclusively Pumping Log

Date: ___/___/___

Pumping Log	
Time of Pump	Amount Pumped
Total Ounces Pumped: _____ oz	

Feeding Log	
Time of Feed	Amount Fed
Total Ounces Fed: _____ oz	

Amount in the freezer at the start of the day: _____ oz
Amount thawed to feed the baby today: − _____ oz
Amount added to the freezer today: + _____ oz
Amount in freezer stash at the end of the day: = _____ oz

Notes: _____
_____
_____
_____
_____
_____
_____

Exclusively Pumping Log

Date:___/___/___

| Pumping Log || Feeding Log ||
Time of Pump	Amount Pumped	Time of Feed	Amount Fed

Total Ounces Pumped: _____ oz Total Ounces Fed: _____ oz

Amount in the freezer at the start of the day: _____ oz
Amount thawed to feed the baby today: -- _____ oz
Amount added to the freezer today: + _____ oz
Amount in freezer stash at the end of the day: = _____ oz

Notes: _____
_____
_____
_____
_____
_____

Exclusively Pumping Log

Date: ___/___/___

Pumping Log		Feeding Log	
Time of Pump	Amount Pumped	Time of Feed	Amount Fed
Total Ounces Pumped: _____ oz		Total Ounces Fed: _____ oz	

Amount in the freezer at the start of the day: _____ oz
Amount thawed to feed the baby today: -- _____ oz
Amount added to the freezer today: + _____ oz
Amount in freezer stash at the end of the day: = _____ oz

Notes: _____
_____
_____
_____
_____
_____
_____

Exclusively Pumping Log

Date: ___/___/___

Pumping Log	
Time of Pump	Amount Pumped
Total Ounces Pumped: _____ oz	

Feeding Log	
Time of Feed	Amount Fed
Total Ounces Fed: _____ oz	

Amount in the freezer at the start of the day: _____ oz
Amount thawed to feed the baby today: −_____ oz
Amount added to the freezer today: +_____ oz
Amount in freezer stash at the end of the day: = _____ oz

Notes: _____
_____
_____
_____
_____
_____

Exclusively Pumping Log

Date: ___/___/___

Pumping Log			Feeding Log	
Time of Pump	Amount Pumped		Time of Feed	Amount Fed
Total Ounces Pumped: _____ oz			Total Ounces Fed: _____ oz	

Amount in the freezer at the start of the day: _____ oz
Amount thawed to feed the baby today: -- _____ oz
Amount added to the freezer today: + _____ oz
Amount in freezer stash at the end of the day: = _____ oz

Notes: _____
_____
_____
_____
_____
_____
_____

Exclusively Pumping Log

Date: ___/___/___

Pumping Log			Feeding Log	
Time of Pump	Amount Pumped		Time of Feed	Amount Fed
Total Ounces Pumped: _____ oz			Total Ounces Fed: _____ oz	

Amount in the freezer at the start of the day: _____ oz
Amount thawed to feed the baby today: -- _____ oz
Amount added to the freezer today: + _____ oz
Amount in freezer stash at the end of the day: = _____ oz

Notes: _____
_____
_____
_____
_____
_____
_____

Exclusively Pumping Log

Date: __/__/__

Pumping Log

Time of Pump	Amount Pumped

Total Ounces Pumped: _____ oz

Feeding Log

Time of Feed	Amount Fed

Total Ounces Fed: _____ oz

Amount in the freezer at the start of the day: _____ oz
Amount thawed to feed the baby today: − _____ oz
Amount added to the freezer today: + _____ oz
Amount in freezer stash at the end of the day: = _____ oz

Notes: _____
_____
_____
_____
_____
_____
_____
_____

Exclusively Pumping Log

Date: ___/___/___

Pumping Log		Feeding Log	
Time of Pump	Amount Pumped	Time of Feed	Amount Fed
Total Ounces Pumped: _____ oz		Total Ounces Fed: _____ oz	

Amount in the freezer at the start of the day: _____ oz
Amount thawed to feed the baby today: -- _____ oz
Amount added to the freezer today: + _____ oz
Amount in freezer stash at the end of the day: = _____ oz

Notes: _____
_____
_____
_____
_____
_____

Exclusively Pumping Log

Date: ___/___/___

Pumping Log			Feeding Log	
Time of Pump	Amount Pumped	Time of Feed	Amount Fed
Total Ounces Pumped: _____ oz		Total Ounces Fed: _____ oz	

Amount in the freezer at the start of the day: _____ oz
Amount thawed to feed the baby today: -- _____ oz
Amount added to the freezer today: + _____ oz
Amount in freezer stash at the end of the day: = _____ oz

Notes: _____
_____
_____
_____
_____
_____
_____

Exclusively Pumping Log

Date: ___/___/___

| Pumping Log || Feeding Log ||
Time of Pump	Amount Pumped	Time of Feed	Amount Fed

Total Ounces Pumped: _____ oz   Total Ounces Fed: _____ oz

Amount in the freezer at the start of the day: _____ oz
Amount thawed to feed the baby today: -- _____ oz
Amount added to the freezer today: + _____ oz
Amount in freezer stash at the end of the day: = _____ oz

Notes: _____
_____
_____
_____
_____
_____
_____

Exclusively Pumping Log

Date: ___/___/___

Pumping Log			Feeding Log	
Time of Pump	**Amount Pumped**		**Time of Feed**	**Amount Fed**
Total Ounces Pumped: _____ oz			Total Ounces Fed: _____ oz	

Amount in the freezer at the start of the day: _____ oz
Amount thawed to feed the baby today: −_____ oz
Amount added to the freezer today: +_____ oz
Amount in freezer stash at the end of the day: =_____ oz

Notes: _____
_____
_____
_____
_____
_____
_____
_____

Exclusively Pumping Log

Date: ___/___/___

| Pumping Log || Feeding Log ||
Time of Pump	Amount Pumped	Time of Feed	Amount Fed
Total Ounces Pumped: _____ oz		Total Ounces Fed: _____ oz	

Amount in the freezer at the start of the day: _____ oz
Amount thawed to feed the baby today: -- _____ oz
Amount added to the freezer today: + _____ oz
Amount in freezer stash at the end of the day: = _____ oz

Notes: _____
_____
_____
_____
_____
_____
_____

Exclusively Pumping Log

Date: ___/___/___

Pumping Log		Feeding Log	
Time of Pump	Amount Pumped	Time of Feed	Amount Fed
Total Ounces Pumped: _____ oz		Total Ounces Fed: _____ oz	

Amount in the freezer at the start of the day: _____ oz
Amount thawed to feed the baby today: − _____ oz
Amount added to the freezer today: + _____ oz
Amount in freezer stash at the end of the day: = _____ oz

Notes: _____
_____
_____
_____
_____
_____

Exclusively Pumping Log

Date: ___/___/___

Pumping Log			Feeding Log	
Time of Pump	Amount Pumped		Time of Feed	Amount Fed
Total Ounces Pumped: _____ oz			Total Ounces Fed: _____ oz	

Amount in the freezer at the start of the day: _____ oz
Amount thawed to feed the baby today: -- _____ oz
Amount added to the freezer today: + _____ oz
Amount in freezer stash at the end of the day: = _____ oz

Notes: _____
_____
_____
_____
_____
_____
_____
_____

Exclusively Pumping Log

Date: ___/___/___

| Pumping Log || Feeding Log ||
Time of Pump	Amount Pumped	Time of Feed	Amount Fed

Total Ounces Pumped: _____ oz   Total Ounces Fed: _____ oz

Amount in the freezer at the start of the day: _____ oz
Amount thawed to feed the baby today: − _____ oz
Amount added to the freezer today: + _____ oz
Amount in freezer stash at the end of the day: = _____ oz

Notes: _____
_____
_____
_____
_____
_____
_____

Exclusively Pumping Log

Date: ___/___/___

Pumping Log			Feeding Log	
Time of Pump	Amount Pumped		Time of Feed	Amount Fed
Total Ounces Pumped: _____ oz			Total Ounces Fed: _____ oz	

Amount in the freezer at the start of the day: _____ oz
Amount thawed to feed the baby today: -- _____ oz
Amount added to the freezer today: + _____ oz
Amount in freezer stash at the end of the day: = _____ oz

Notes: _____
_____
_____
_____
_____
_____
_____
_____

Exclusively Pumping Log

Date:___/___/___

Pumping Log		Feeding Log	
Time of Pump	Amount Pumped	Time of Feed	Amount Fed
Total Ounces Pumped: _____ oz		Total Ounces Fed: _____ oz	

Amount in the freezer at the start of the day: _____ oz
Amount thawed to feed the baby today: −_____ oz
Amount added to the freezer today: +_____ oz
Amount in freezer stash at the end of the day: =_____ oz

Notes: _____
_____
_____
_____
_____
_____
_____

Exclusively Pumping Log

Date: __/__/__

Pumping Log		Feeding Log	
Time of Pump	Amount Pumped	Time of Feed	Amount Fed
Total Ounces Pumped: _____ oz		Total Ounces Fed: _____ oz	

Amount in the freezer at the start of the day: _____ oz
Amount thawed to feed the baby today: -- _____ oz
Amount added to the freezer today: + _____ oz
Amount in freezer stash at the end of the day: = _____ oz

Notes: _____
_____
_____
_____
_____
_____
_____

Exclusively Pumping Log

Date: __/__/__

Pumping Log ||	Feeding Log	
Time of Pump	Amount Pumped	Time of Feed	Amount Fed

Total Ounces Pumped: _____ oz   Total Ounces Fed: _____ oz

Amount in the freezer at the start of the day: _____ oz
Amount thawed to feed the baby today: -- _____ oz
Amount added to the freezer today: + _____ oz
Amount in freezer stash at the end of the day: = _____ oz

Notes: _____
_____
_____
_____
_____
_____
_____
_____

Exclusively Pumping Log

Date: ___/___/___

Pumping Log		Feeding Log	
Time of Pump	**Amount Pumped**	**Time of Feed**	**Amount Fed**
Total Ounces Pumped: _____ oz		Total Ounces Fed: _____ oz	

Amount in the freezer at the start of the day: _____ oz
Amount thawed to feed the baby today: −_____ oz
Amount added to the freezer today: +_____ oz
Amount in freezer stash at the end of the day: =_____ oz

Notes: _____
_____
_____
_____
_____
_____

Exclusively Pumping Log

Date: ___/___/___

Pumping Log			Feeding Log	
Time of Pump	**Amount Pumped**	**Time of Feed**	**Amount Fed**
Total Ounces Pumped: _____ oz		Total Ounces Fed: _____ oz	

Amount in the freezer at the start of the day: _____ oz
Amount thawed to feed the baby today: − _____ oz
Amount added to the freezer today: + _____ oz
Amount in freezer stash at the end of the day: = _____ oz

Notes: _____
_____
_____
_____
_____
_____

Exclusively Pumping Log

Date: ___/___/___

Pumping Log	
Time of Pump	Amount Pumped
Total Ounces Pumped: _____ oz	

Feeding Log	
Time of Feed	Amount Fed
Total Ounces Fed: _____ oz	

Amount in the freezer at the start of the day: _____ oz
Amount thawed to feed the baby today: -- _____ oz
Amount added to the freezer today: + _____ oz
Amount in freezer stash at the end of the day: = _____ oz

Notes: _____
_____
_____
_____
_____
_____
_____

Exclusively Pumping Log

Date: ___/___/___

Pumping Log			Feeding Log	
Time of Pump	Amount Pumped	Time of Feed	Amount Fed

Total Ounces Pumped: _____ oz   Total Ounces Fed: _____ oz

Amount in the freezer at the start of the day: _____ oz
Amount thawed to feed the baby today: -- _____ oz
Amount added to the freezer today: + _____ oz
Amount in freezer stash at the end of the day: = _____ oz

Notes: _____
_____
_____
_____
_____
_____
_____

Exclusively Pumping Log

Date: ___/___/___

Pumping Log		Feeding Log	
Time of Pump	**Amount Pumped**	**Time of Feed**	**Amount Fed**
Total Ounces Pumped: _____ oz		**Total Ounces Fed:** _____ oz	

Amount in the freezer at the start of the day: _____ oz
Amount thawed to feed the baby today: -- _____ oz
Amount added to the freezer today: + _____ oz
Amount in freezer stash at the end of the day: = _____ oz

Notes: _____
_____
_____
_____
_____
_____

Exclusively Pumping Log

Date: ___/___/___

Pumping Log

Time of Pump	Amount Pumped
Total Ounces Pumped: _____	oz

Feeding Log

Time of Feed	Amount Fed
Total Ounces Fed: _____	oz

Amount in the freezer at the start of the day: _____ oz
Amount thawed to feed the baby today: −_____ oz
Amount added to the freezer today: +_____ oz
Amount in freezer stash at the end of the day: =_____ oz

Notes: _____
_____
_____
_____
_____
_____
_____

Exclusively Pumping Log

Date: ___/___/___

Pumping Log			Feeding Log	
Time of Pump	Amount Pumped		Time of Feed	Amount Fed
Total Ounces Pumped: _____ oz			Total Ounces Fed: _____ oz	

Amount in the freezer at the start of the day: _____ oz
Amount thawed to feed the baby today: -- _____ oz
Amount added to the freezer today: + _____ oz
Amount in freezer stash at the end of the day: = _____ oz

Notes: _____
_____
_____
_____
_____
_____
_____

Exclusively Pumping Log

Date: __/__/__

Pumping Log		Feeding Log	
Time of Pump	Amount Pumped	Time of Feed	Amount Fed
Total Ounces Pumped: _____ oz		Total Ounces Fed: _____ oz	

Amount in the freezer at the start of the day: _____ oz
Amount thawed to feed the baby today: -- _____ oz
Amount added to the freezer today: + _____ oz
Amount in freezer stash at the end of the day: = _____ oz

Notes: _____
_____
_____
_____
_____
_____
_____
_____

Exclusively Pumping Log

Date: ___/___/___

Pumping Log			Feeding Log	
Time of Pump	Amount Pumped		Time of Feed	Amount Fed

Total Ounces Pumped: _____ oz   Total Ounces Fed: _____ oz

Amount in the freezer at the start of the day: _____ oz
Amount thawed to feed the baby today: −_____ oz
Amount added to the freezer today: +_____ oz
Amount in freezer stash at the end of the day: =_____ oz

Notes: _____
_____
_____
_____
_____
_____

Exclusively Pumping Log

Date:___/___/___

Pumping Log			Feeding Log	
Time of Pump	Amount Pumped		Time of Feed	Amount Fed
Total Ounces Pumped: _____ oz			Total Ounces Fed: _____ oz	

Amount in the freezer at the start of the day: _____ oz
Amount thawed to feed the baby today: -- _____ oz
Amount added to the freezer today: + _____ oz
Amount in freezer stash at the end of the day: = _____ oz

Notes: _____
_____
_____
_____
_____
_____

Made in the USA
Coppell, TX
29 September 2023